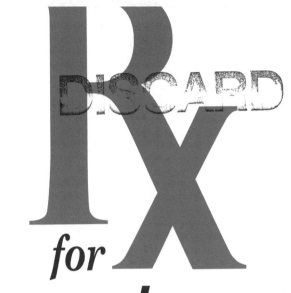

RX

for
computer eyes

proven ways
to prevent

and correct

the eye strain

caused by

modern life

by

427768

Kevin D. Geiger, O.D.

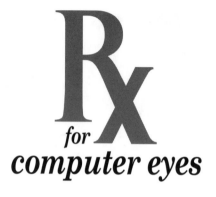

computer eyes

proven ways
to prevent
and correct
the eye strain
caused by
modern life

by
Kevin D. Geiger, O.D.

edited by
W.W. Pratt

Printed in the USA

ISBN 1884820-81-6
978-1-884820-81-6
LCC # 2005934925

Safe Goods/ ATN Publishing
561 Shunpike Rd., Sheffield, MA 01257
413-229-7935
www.safegoodspub.com

Table of Contents

Foreword

Do you know you are not supposed to become more and more nearsighted, year after year, after the eyes stop growing? Are you one of the millions of Americans whose eyesight continues to worsen every year or so? Did you receive your first eyeglass prescription for nearsightedness after the age of 18? Would you like to discover ways to use your eyes as they were intended and thwart further compromises to your vision?

If you answered "Yes!" to any of these four questions, then you need to read this book! This book will detail the events that cause one's nearsightedness to get progressively worse, and simple steps to prevent or slowdown this process.

I chose the title *Rx for Computer Eyes* for this book because, despite the fact that many people believe the computer screen is a beneficial part of modern life, it certainly isn't when it comes to their vision. I'll say it as plainly and simply as I can: "taking advantage of all the speed and convenience of a modern computer may be good for your pursuits and your pocketbook, but not for your precious eyes."

This book, then, is a "must read" for every computer user, be they high school, college or postgraduate student, business person or scientist, computer gaming enthusiast, dedicated emailer, cyber-shopper, and everyone else – whether they ever touch a computer or not – who spends many hours each day doing close visual work.

Do I say this because I want to sell you this book? No (even though I do hope you will take the time to read and learn from it). I say it because I have spent my career finding ways to help people retain and improve their vision. Once you finish it, it is my sincere hope – and my full expectation – that you will take away with you these "proven ways to prevent and correct the eye strain caused by modern life."

Now let's begin …

Chapter One:
In The Beginning

When mankind first found his way onto this earth, whether your personal beliefs lean toward divine creationism or Darwin's theory of evolution, we were not meant to focus our vision intently on a single, flat plane for extended periods of time. Our ancestors were simple hunters and gatherers, whose very existence demanded they watch all the things in their environment, near and far. There were no books, no computers, no desk work to be done. Instead, the tasks early man needed to perform – stalking game, finding edible plants, searching out shelter from the harsh elements, cooking and eating, raising the young – were all performed in relatively short periods of time, certainly well below thirty minutes for any single task.

Many studies over the years have supported my contention that "prolonged near work can lead to the development (and progression) of myopia." Below I would like to highlight three of these studies.

The first study, done by Dr. F. Young, et al, and reported in *The American Journal of Optometry and Archives of the American Academy of Optometry* in 1969, took place in Barrow, Alaska. Young and his associates set out to test the genetic theory of myopia (nearsightedness). The Eskimo population was a unique group to study because the older generation was essentially illiterate and had never gone through formal schooling. Their children, on the other hand, were the first generation to go through school. The older generation lived a typical outdoor Eskimo life of hunting and fishing, with little close work. The younger generation, however, did a great deal more close work because of reading and other school-related nearpoint work. Despite the sharp contrast in nearpoint activities, if myopia was indeed hereditary, the rate of myopia in the children and in the parents should be similar, (if not identical). Yet the results of the study are quite amazing, as the following results show. Of the 130 parents, 128 had excellent distance vision (no myopia) and only two were myopic. Of those two, one parent had one step of myopia (0.25 Diopters) and the other, who was the tribal record keeper, had six steps of myopia (1.50 Diopters). What about their children? Six out of ten (a full 60 percent) of the children were myopic. The genetic theory of myopia cannot explain this, and since both groups essentially ate the same diet, the differences in the rates of myopia cannot be explained away by nutritional differences.

Young concluded that long periods spent reading school work by the younger generation was the cause of their increased rate of myopia. Following this study, Young set out to prove this environment-induced myopia theory. He tested his theory using chimpanzees in a laboratory setting because their eyes are very similar to human eyes. In the laboratory, he was able to restrict the vision of the chimpanzees so that they could not see further than fifteen inches, similar to a person doing hours of reading or computer work. Obviously, these chimpanzees were allowed no distance vision at all, and it is important to note that chimps living in the wild are never nearsighted. The result was that after a few months of testing, Young's laboratory chimpanzees *did develop myopia!*

In another important study published in *The American Journal of Optometry* in 1980, Drs. J. Kinney, S. Laria and A. Ryan, et al, were able to show that members of submarine crews will have increases in myopia after doing a tour of duty due to the restricted viewing distances inside submarines.

Many more studies *clearly* demonstrate that prolonged close activities can and will lead to increased myopia. I will tell you what I often tell my patients, "Don't change your job. Don't avoid studying. Change your habits!" The suggestions later in this book such as frequent rest breaks looking far away, doing near-far focusing exercises, along with other eye exercises and/ or reading glasses can help to prevent or reduce increases in myopia. The prolonged time we spend on "near" tasks, such as reading and computer use, in our daily lives – one hour, two hours, eight hours – at any one sitting is very stressful to our visual system. Words and numbers on a printed page or a computer screen are not the three dimensional objects for which our eyes and the process of vision were designed. Likewise, how much of the activities we perform for our livings and for our hobbies – tying a perfect fly for trout fishing, building scale models, lovingly crocheting a very special blanket for a newborn grandchild – demand that we concentrate on visual items at one distance for long periods of time?

We were meant to vary our visual focus constantly, looking from one object to another in rapid succession. Yet prolonged near tasks and two-dimensional near task focus on detailed handiwork, books, spread sheets, text and computer images, are at the root of today's modern, information-age society. Of all of these, the computer screen is the worst offender of all for the health and functionality of our eyes because the images are made-up of pixels which cause the letters to flicker and float on the monitor screen, adding an even greater stress to our visual system. Studies show that our focusing systems are confused from the pixels "floating" in space and our eyes do not accurately focus on them; the quality of letters on a computer screen are not as clear as words on a printed page. In Chapter 6, "Computers and the Eyes," I will further detail the many problems computers cause for our eyes and give you explicit, easy to implement changes you can immediately make to improve your comfort at your computer workstation.

Chapter Two:
The Basic Eye

Author's Note: Before beginning this chapter, take two minutes to look away from the page – as far away as you can – and focus on several different objects at least 20 feet away. Even better if you can turn your attention for that time to an object in motion. Then repeat this exercise for another 60 seconds each and every time you start a new chapter in this book. This is how human eyes are meant to be used, and how they will stay well conditioned for the clearest and most comfortable vision possible.

It is important to any discussion of how to improve and preserve your vision that you understand the construction and function of the complicated organ we call the eyeball. This chapter will give you that sort of "thumb nail" explanation of the human eye and how it works. While it may appear overly simple and somewhat boring initially, please know that it is the information your eye care professional begins with, and the information that will help you, immeasurably, in learning how to care for your eyes, especially when you use them in the stress-filled environment of the computer screen.

A good starting point is how our eyes change from birth, through our teen years, and into adulthood (see Figure 1). Our eyes

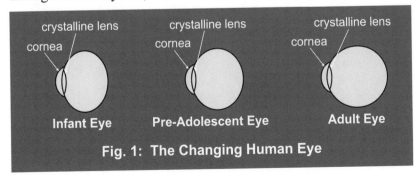

Fig. 1: The Changing Human Eye

change shape and functionality many times during our lives. Understanding those changes is the key to discovering ways to preserve our precious vision throughout the years of our lives.

When we humans are born, our eyes have a limited focusing power. We don't really need any more critical focus, since our world revolves around our family – principally our mothers or other substitute care-givers – who do the serious "looking" for the needs and hazards our young lives require. As we grow from infants to children and then into preadolescent years, our eyeball grows from its short oval shape to a more rounded sphere capable of better focusing light passing through the front of our eyes and being refracted into images we can interpret as the "things" we actually see. As we grow and mature to adulthood, the eyeball continues to elongate from the cornea to the retina at the rear of the organ, leaving us with what we will know as our adult vision.

The essence about what we call adult vision lies principally in the *refractive power* of the eye. This refractive power is the combined focusing ability of the cornea and the crystalline lens, yet as infants and children it is usually too weak to focus the rays of light from a distant object onto the retina unless the lens of the eye flexes (focuses).

When we are fully grown, the power of the eyes we were born with is now just right. Now the lens does not have to flex (focus) to get the image of a distant object sharply focused on the retina. This is the sort of uncorrected vision nature intended for us. In this normal, or *emmetropic* eye, as depicted in Figure 2, parallel rays of light (from an object 20 feet away or greater) enter your eye through the cornea. The cornea

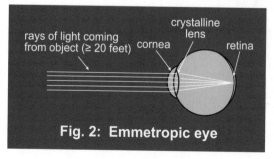

Fig. 2: Emmetropic eye

and lens work in combination, without having to flex the crystalline lens to focus these parallel rays precisely to a point of light on the retina at the back surface of the eye. Unfortunately for many of us, the emmetropic (or "perfect" vision) of our adolescence does not stay with us nearly long enough. Many of us cannot enjoy the benefits of this type of vision without corrective aids. This is where eye care professionals – optometrists, ophthalmologists – and the individual himself or herself must step in and affect changes to our optics.

Figure 3, right, illustrates one of the most common anomalies of the human eye, *myopia* or *nearsightedness*. When those parallel rays of light (the image) enter the eye, the cornea and lens have too much refractive power for the

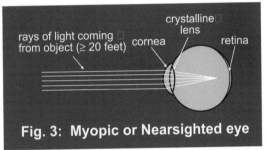

Fig. 3: Myopic or Nearsighted eye

length of the eye, and thus focus the light (image) in front of the retina. The result is a blurred, out of focus image reaching the retina and the brain. Eye care professionals can easily correct this by prescribing a "minus" lens that diverges the light rays, causing the image to be shifted further back onto the retina.

Figure 4 illustrates the opposite condition, the hyperopic or farsighted eye. Here, the cornea and lens combine to deliver too little refractive power power for the length of the eye and, therefore, are unable to focus the image closely

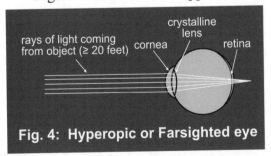

Fig. 4: Hyperopic or Farsighted eye

enough to project a crisp, clear image on the retina. The image this eye sees is actually focused just behind the eye structure.

A "plus" lens can correct this by converging the image forward onto the retina.

There is a third and equally common abnormality in our vision – the astigmatic eye. The word astigma literally means an image without stigma or point. Therefore, the parallel rays of light are not focused at a single point, but rather at two points. Unfortunately, the retina needs a perfectly focused point in order for the image to be seen clearly. A simple minus or plus lens cannot correct this condition. When astigmatism is present, a lens must have two powers, corresponding to where the two points of light are actually focused by the eye. The optics related to astigmatism can assume any of five corrective scenarios.

Most astigmatic vision can be corrected through the use of a variety of lens styles and/or combinations. These are: (1) both minus power lenses; (2) both plus power lenses; (3) one minus lens, one plus lens; (4) only a minus power lens in a certain meridian; or, (5) only a plus power lens in a certain meridian. Cases (4) and (5) would occur if one point was focused on

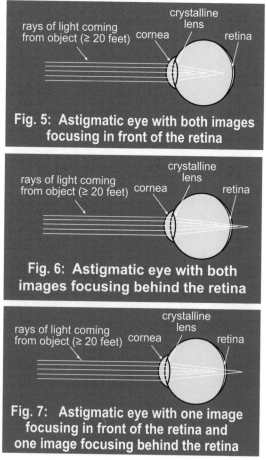

Fig. 5: Astigmatic eye with both images focusing in front of the retina

Fig. 6: Astigmatic eye with both images focusing behind the retina

Fig. 7: Astigmatic eye with one image focusing in front of the retina and one image focusing behind the retina

the retina and the other point either in front of the retina, as in scenario (4), or behind the retina, as in scenario (5).

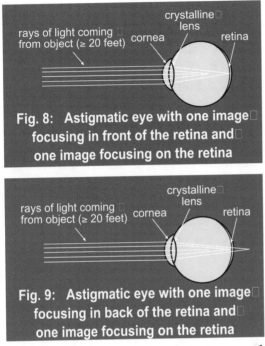

Fig. 8: **Astigmatic eye with one image focusing in front of the retina and one image focusing on the retina**

Fig. 9: **Astigmatic eye with one image focusing in back of the retina and one image focusing on the retina**

There is one other vision condition that is no less troubling to those whom it afflicts. *Presbyopia* can occur in eyes with no refractive errors, as well as to myopic, hyperopic and astigmatic eyes. Presbyopia is the condition that can affect us, usually between ages 40 and 45, to need reading glasses or bifocals. Without getting into too much detail, as we age the crystalline lens in our eye will lose its ability to flex when it is focusing. When we look at objects closer than 20 feet, the lens must focus (flex) in order for the object to be clearly focused on the retina. This is similar to viewing objects through a camera lens. If the camera is focused on an object that is 20 feet away, any objects closer than 20 feet will not be clear through the camera lens. In order for us to view these closer objects clearly, we would have to "focus" the camera lens. This is what happens with the lens in our eyes. Unfortunately, with age, the lens cannot adjust to focus as much, nor as easily, as in our earlier years. The reason why reading or viewing of a computer screen is generally affected first is because these are both done at such a close distance (usually about 16 inches) and require a very large amount of focusing on the part of the lens. The closer the object is to you, the greater the amount of focusing will be required.

This is where corrective lenses come into play. With nearsightedness, or myopia, the eyeball is too long from cornea to retina for its refractive power (i.e., the focusing power is too strong for the length of the eyeball). This may be apparent at birth, or it may present itself several years down the road as the eye grows towards maturity. The answer is a corrective lens that can move the focal point into contact with the retina.

The farsighted, or hyperopic eye, is characterized by refractive power that never developed sufficiently to focus light rays entering through the cornea and lens onto the retina, even as the eye developed, or that the eyeball was too short in length. Here again, corrective lenses can be prescribed that will bring images into clear focus.

As stated earlier, nature intended for all human eyes to be *farsighted at birth* and as the individual grows to become more and more nearsighted until emmetropic ("perfect") vision can be realized after the eyes stop growing. Now that the eyes have stopped growing, they should no longer be farsighted; they should not be nearsighted; they should be perfect. This is why many eye doctors will tell parents of slightly farsighted children that their child "may grow out of this" or that their eyes "will get better." Unfortunately for nearsighted children, their eyesight will only get worse as they grow. This is why I tell my young myopic patients that their prescriptions will probably have to get stronger and stronger as they grow older.

I am sure that many nearsighted people will read this and say, "but I was in college when I got my first pair of glasses," or "my prescription has changed every year from age 22 to 35!" It is for these people and the millions of others with similar experiences that this book has been written! Nature did not plan on these occurrences! Any progression or "start" of nearsightedness in the twenties or later is not a natural progression;

it is a direct result of your reading/viewing habits and your environment! *I cannot stress this point enough!* How you pursue your near-distance viewing tasks is the cause of this; your myopia will continue to grow more severe, unless you change your ways. So then, I offer this most sincere advice to you: *Do not change jobs – change your habits!*

Chapter Three:
So What's Going On?

Author's Note: Ah, ah, ah! Remember, before you begin this chapter, take time to look away from the page, as far away as you can, and focus on several distant objects. Your eyes will thank you for the break from near-distance strain.

Anyone who spends many hours, regularly, performing close or near work will experience changes in their vision. Changes will include any or all: headaches, eyestrain, progression of nearsightedness. That's a hard fact that none of us can escape. Near activities include computer activities, reading, deskwork, sewing and needlepoint, hobby crafts and the like.

Humans were not meant to perform near tasks for lengthy periods of time, regularly. When you wear corrective lenses (eyeglasses or contact lenses), the prescription will focus the image of an object at 20 feet onto the retina with no focusing by the crystalline lens of the eye. (The focusing system of the eye, therefore, is relaxed and not having to strain to inform you what it is seeing). Even if you are not farsighted and do not need a distance prescription, you will be exerting no effort when viewing objects at 20 feet or further.

Any object closer than 20 feet, however, requires the eyes to work at focusing. Think of a camera. If the camera is focused at an object that is 20 feet away, any object closer than that will tend to be out of focus and blurry. You would have to refocus the camera, therefore, to whatever distance the near object was located at in order for its image to be clear. The human eye is basically the same. For the perfect 20/20 person, or the individual that wears distance glasses and has *corrected* 20/20 vision at distance, his eyes would have to work (focus) just a little to see an object at 19 feet clearly … a little bit more for an object at

18 feet ... a little more still for an object at 17 feet ... etc. ... until about 20 to 24 inches for his computer screen or about 16 or 18 inches for his book or desk papers. This is a *large* effort for his eyes. Despite the work they must do, the eyes can handle this for a while. It is the constant long periods of very close work, day after day, that will begin to take its toll on one's visual system. Think of any other muscle in your body. Can you clench your fist tightly and hold it for 15 minutes ... 30 minutes ... two hours? How would it feel after you've flexed it for a very long time? Try this experiment. Make a very tight fist and hold it for 30 seconds. When you are done, open your hand. It's difficult, isn't it? Notice how your hand wants to stay in that clenched position? The same holds true for the human eyes. If you "flex" your eye muscles for a very long time, they have a hard time returning to a fully relaxed state. Remember, a fully relaxed state enables you (either with corrective lenses or without) to see objects clearly at 20 feet. However, after many days, then weeks, then months of performing near-point tasks for an extended period of time, (e.g., computer operation or programming six hours a day, five days a week) instead of your eyes relaxing and focusing to 20 feet, they will eventually only relax and focus to 19 feet. If you continue to do a lot of near-point work for another couple of months, your eyes might only relax and focus to 18 feet. *This process will surely continue unless you take charge and change your habits.* This process can sometimes be reversed, if it is not too late. If an individual's eyes are "embedded" in nearsightedness, though, it is usually too late.

We will now turn our attention to slowing down the progression of diminishing vision and preventing further changes to the eyes in the future. Unfortunately, this is how human eyes deal with the "nearpoint stress." There are three ways your eyes will handle excessive reading or computer work, day in and day out. You will very likely experience headaches, eyestrain or increased nearsightedness.

Obviously, as individuals, the progression of nearsighted-ness and its symptoms will affect each of us at differing rates and to differing degrees. I cannot predict whether this will occur in two months, six months or a year, so begin now to change your habits in order to lessen the tremendous strain you are exerting on your vision.

Chapter Four:
Change Your Habits

Author's Note: Hey, doctor's orders! Put down this book for two minutes, look away from the page, relax your eyes, and build better eye health for yourself. Why not, when it is so easy to do? The key to avoid weakening of your vision caused by all that endless paperwork and hours peering into a computer monitor is to change how you approach those tasks.

Following a few simple and practical suggestions is a must for anyone required (or personally motivated) to engage in prolonged close work. First, have your eyes examined right away if it's been more than a year since your last eye exam. This seems logical, but we all tend to put off routine annual eye examinations. Anyone wearing eyeglasses or contact lenses should be seen annually, not just to check their prescription, but also the health of their eyes.

The retina is the only place in the body where we can observe arteries and veins at the same time, without doing any cutting. Often, many diseases or disorders that affect our vascular system can be detected during a routine eye examination – i.e., diabetes, hypertension, AIDS, systemic lupus erythematous, sickle cell anemia. Sometimes, even the care we give the rest of our body can put our vision at risk. Many oral prescription drugs can cause changes to our eyes. Prednisone, chloroquine, tamoxifen are a few drugs that require a thorough eye examination, at least once a year. It is always best to check with your internist, because some drugs do require even more frequent eye examinations.

Before going any further, I would like to make it perfectly clear, too, that *all eye examinations are not created equal!* I recommend you see an eye doctor that will test not only if you can see clearly up close, but how your eyes work while performing near tasks. And remember, *not all eye doctors* probe how their patient's eyes work while performing near tasks.

How can you be sure that your eye doctor will probe how your eyes work when you read or do other near tasks? Truthfully, it is not an easy task. The best way (although, certainly, not the only way) is to seek an optometrist or ophthalmologist who specializes in doing vision therapy (eye exercises). These eye doctors routinely probe their patients' eye coordination and eye teaming when they examine their eyes. If they have the designation FCOVD after their name, they are a Fellow of the College of Optometrists in Vision Development. This is an organization of optometrists that are certified in "behavioral" optometry. These eye doctors gear their practices towards probing for eye coordination problems, eye focusing problems as well as general eye care.

Just because an optometrist does not have the FCOVD designation after their name does not mean that they do not check for eye focusing or eye coordination problems. I, for instance, am not a fellow of COVD, but I am more than qualified to diagnose and help in many instances where there are eye focusing or eye coordination problems. I am a past recipient of the Frederick Brock Memorial Award from the State University of New York, State College of Optometry. This was granted to me in recognition of my skills and knowledge in eye coordination and eye teaming problems, as well as other areas in which an individual's eyes are not working adequately and efficiently for that person to correctly perceive and use the images that the eyes are seeing. (I no longer treat these individuals; my practice is not geared towards eye exercises and vision therapy, and so I never pursued a fellowship from COVD.)

I suggest seeking out an FCOVD optometrist simply because it is the easiest way for you to find an eye care professional who specializes in and gears his or her practice towards eye coordination and eye focusing problems and probes for them during the exam process. The COVD's contact information (www.covd.org) will help you locate an FCOVD optometrist in your area. (The Optometric Extension Program, www.oep.org, is also an excellent resource to find behavioral optometrists.) After your eye examination, you will either be given an eyeglass prescription for your near tasks, vision therapy eye exercises, both ... or, best of all, simply a "clean bill of health."

Now, let's take some time to examine what you can do, yourself, to improve your eye health and function. Here is where you can be your own best "doctor" for vision. After any near-distance tasks (computer, sewing, reading, etc.) for fifteen minutes, you need to stop and take a two minute rest break. Remember, we are not meant to read for prolonged periods of time. Your two-minute break should consist of looking at a clock on the wall, at a sign out the window, kids playing outside or passersby going about their business. Focus your look at least ten feet away, ideally 20 feet or more, and focus on something ... not just a blank wall.

If you feel yourself getting tense, tight or "cramped," perform deep breathing exercises and stretching as needed. Many of you who are reading this perform near-tasks for extended periods of time, and you must consciously decide to do the above. Remember the explanation that looking at close work will "flex" your eyes' focusing muscles, and looking far away will relax them? Then it only makes sense that reading or performing other near-point tasks for extended periods of time *must* be broken up at regular intervals. Make it a personal regimen to stop close work every fifteen minutes and take this two-minute break.

After an hour, you *must* get up, go to the bathroom, get a drink of water, whatever – *don't* sit at your desk or near point activity for more than one hour! Humans are not meant to sit or stay in one position for extended periods of time. We need to move. Movement is essential. If you are doing prolonged near work,

Movement is essential. If you are doing prolonged near work, you *must* continue to take the two-minute rest break after every fifteen minutes, and do the get up/stretch/walk around/exercise after each hour of work. By the way, if you are worried about taking breaks from the computer or paperwork in your workplace, don't be. Employers today are becoming very informed about occupational hazards, including threats to workers' vision. By taking the breaks cited above, you will actually be a better employee – not worse. You will be more comfortable, and therefore happier and more efficient! (Tell this to your boss or supervisor and say that you are following doctor's orders!)

Chapter Five:
Calisthenics For Your Eyes

Author's Note: Once again, dear readers, take two minutes right now to rest your over-flexed eyes, because what you are about to read will surely give you a work-out to save your sight.

I think by now we are all in agreement that modern day life and work puts an incredible strain on the ability of our eyes to "flex" in order to focus properly. In order to deal with the great demand and strain on our eyes, we all need to exercise and tone up the muscles of our eyes if we are going to preserve our vision. That's where what I like to call "eye calisthenics" comes into play.

The following exercises can help those of you who must perform near-distance tasks for three hours or more a day, three or more days a week. Try each of them, and see the difference in how you feel and how you see.

Before I explain the exercises, I want to stress two very important "must dos" whenever you are doing prolonged near tasks: first, you must remember to breathe in order to ease the stress your eyes and body feel with prolonged near work; and, second, make it a point to blink frequently ... the best blink is a soft, gentle movement where you keep your eyes closed for a count of two or three seconds before re-opening. This is a very soothing activity for your eyes.

Near-Far Flexibility Exercise: This is a relatively simple exercise to help keep your focusing system flexible and fluid rather than tight and stiff. All you need for this exercise is your finger and a distant object (20 to 30 feet away). Hold your extended finger – your index finger is usually best – at eye level. You can do this with one eye closed or both eyes open. The closer you hold your finger to your eyes the more difficult this will be. A good starting distance is 16 inches or closer. You should then bring your finger closer and closer to your eyes as you get better and better with this exercise.

To begin, look at your fingerprint on your extended finger trying to focus on your fingerprint as clearly as possible for five seconds. Next, look at a distant object (a clock on the wall, a sign outside the window, etc. ... but not a blank wall) 20 feet away or further. If you are in a confined area, try looking at the farthest object in the room. While 20 feet or further is ideal, any distance more than three feet will still allow you to benefit from this exercise. Again, try to see this object clearly for five seconds. Now, refocus on your fingerprint, getting this clear for five seconds. Repeat this cycle of focusing on your fingerprint for five seconds and then the object for five seconds for a total of about two minutes. You can do this while doing lots of near work to keep your over-focused eye muscles flexible, or, you can do this at your leisure. I often tell my patients to do it at home while watching TV. Commercial breaks on TV are usually for two minutes. Use the commercial breaks to do this near-far exercise for the full two minutes. Repeat this exercise about five times each day.

Another point I make to my patients is to do these exercises five to seven days a week. Remember, doing these exercises every day is best, but doing them six days a week is better than doing them just five days a week, and five days a week is better still than four ... and so on. They are very easy to do – *do them!*

Pencil Push-ups: For this exercise you will need a pen or a pencil. The starting position for this exercise is to hold the pen or pencil about 16 inches in front of your nose. Look at the tip of the pen (pencil). Bring the pen towards your nose slowly while still seeing the tip of the pen clearly. If the pen tip ever becomes double (you see two pen tips) or blurred, stop and move the pen away from your nose to the starting position (16 inches). If you don't see two tips, continue to slowly bring the pen towards your nose until about 1/4 inch from the tip of your nose. Now, slowly move the pen away from your nose to the original starting distance (16 inches). You should repeat this movement of bringing the pen closer and further from your nose for about two minutes. As with the near-far exercise, doing this five times per day, every day each week should be your goal.

Eye Rotations: When we perform near tasks for prolonged periods of time, our eyes are mostly confined to a very limited area of eye movements. The purpose of the eye rotations exercise is to move the eyes or "stretch" the eye muscles. These exercises can be performed either standing or seated.

With your head level and your eyes pointing straight ahead, look up to the ceiling for two to three seconds; next, look down to the floor for two to three seconds. Next, look to the right for two to three seconds and, finally, look to the left for two to three seconds. Be careful when looking in each of the four directions. You must keep your head still, only moving your eyes. Looking in each of these four directions constitutes one full cycle or rotation. Continue these cycles for about two minutes. You can speed up the pace of your eye movements if you prefer not to hold each gaze for the full three seconds.

A variation to the above eye movements can be performed by looking back and forth between two of the gaze directions. For instance, a cycle would consist of looking from left to right and then back to the left. You would look left to right, therefore, and then right to left, repeating these eye movements for about one minute. Next you would do cycles of looking up and down for another minute as well.

Yet another variation to these "stretching" eye movements is circular or clock rotations. Again, seated or standing, with your head level and your eyes looking straight ahead, look at all of the numbers on an imaginary clock. First look up to 12 o'clock, then towards 1 o'clock, then 2 o'clock, then 3 o'clock, etc. until you end up back at 12 o'clock. Look at each of the hours of the clock for about two seconds, or else look at one hour, then the next hour without stopping along the way. Do these forward (clockwise) "clock rotations" for about 30 seconds and then reverse your rotations counter-clockwise for 30 seconds. Repeat the cycle. Perform these rotations for two to five minutes. Do not do these until you are fatigued. Instead, do them until it just starts to feel uncomfortable, or for five minutes, whichever comes first. You can do all three of these eye movement exercises or any combination of them. Remember, frequency and repetition are the basis of physical conditioning. The more often you do them and the more days a week you perform these exercises, the better.

Palming: This is a relaxation exercise that I recommend to many patients who complain that they have a dull ache in their eyes from doing too much near work. This will relax and soothe your eyes and your body. This is done while seated at a desk or table. Sit with your feet flat on the floor. Place your elbows on the table, with the palms of your hands facing you. Lean slightly forward so that your eyes rest fully cupped in the palms of your hands. Your palms should be pressed lightly against the bones just below your eyes. There should be no pressure exerted on the eyes themselves. The four fingers of one hand should lie gently across the four fingers of the other hand on your forehead. You should be very comfortable in this position; if you are not comfortable, you are not in the correct position.

Close your eyes. Breathe deeply. (Deep breathing consists of inhaling through your nose, feeling your chest cavity expand, and exhaling very slowly out of your mouth.) Slow, deep breathing is very important. With your eyes closed, and your hands (palms) preventing outside light from reaching your eyelids, concentrate on a serene, peaceful setting. Imagine yourself at a beach, watching the waves crash on the shore. Imagine you are watching the sunrise or sunset, or imagine whatever it is that will help you to relax. Continue this for as long as you need to relax; usually, anywhere from three to 20 minutes. You should feel refreshed and relaxed after a "palming" session.

Last, but certainly not least, here are some important points to take with you from this chapter:

- Humans are not meant to stay still in any position for prolonged periods of time. In fact, our lymphatic system relies entirely on us moving about in order to do its job properly. American doctors are finally catching on to this. Now, doctors in hospitals are getting patients out of bed as soon as possible after surgery in order to speed up their recovery time. The same holds true for your eyes. They will not be comfortable looking at a constant distance or a confined work area that minimizes eye movements for extended periods of time. The eyes need to move both from near to far and to different gaze angles such as to the right, left, up and down.

- I have been harping on this at the beginning of each chapter of this book, but it bears repeating here again. While doing prolonged near work, take a break every fifteen minutes and give your eyes some needed relaxation by looking far away (10 feet or further) for a full two minutes. Take these two minute breaks every 15 minutes. After one hour, stop and get up. Go to the bathroom, get a drink of water – it doesn't matter what you do, just get up and walk around. Don't sit at your desk for more than one hour straight. Don't worry about your job performance; you will probably be a better employee. You will be more comfortable and therefore, you will be more efficient and happier.

This chapter detailed very easy, no-nonsense exercises that anyone and everyone should do if they spend many hours doing close work. Don't dismiss these suggestions as too easy or not useful. Trust me, *these are a must!*

25

Chapter Six:
Computers and Your Eyes

Author's Note: Now what have we just learned? Right – it's time to rest your eyes once more! Take your two minute break right now.

I would be very surprised if more than 10 percent of all who read this book do not use a computer regularly. Computers are now used by more than 100 million Americans daily at their jobs. Home internet use is skyrocketing too. In fact, it is estimated that even children two to five years old are spending *an average* of 27 minutes in front of a computer monitor every day!

If computers did not cause serious stress for our vision, neck, back and shoulders, there would be no need for this book. Unfortunately, computers are not entirely good for us. As with reading, computers are good for the brain, but not for the eyes. In fact, computers have caused so many complaints by regular users that the American Optometric Association (AOA), has classified a new term, "Computer Vision Syndrome" (CVS).

Computer Vision Syndrome is defined as "the complex of eye and vision problems related to near work experienced during computer use." The symptoms of CVS include:

- eyestrain (sore eyes or eye fatigue)
- headache
- blurred near vision
- slowness in changing the focus of the eyes
- blur in the distance after near work
- glare (light) sensitivity
- eye irritation (burning, dryness, redness)
- contact lens discomfort
- neck and shoulder pain
- back pain
- development of myopia (nearsightedness)

These symptoms are caused by a combination of the limitations of the individual computer user's visual capabilities, poor visual ergonomics and prolonged computer use. Computers are very visually demanding and, therefore, cause CVS complaints by individuals who otherwise would have no such symptoms if performing a less visually demanding task.

The National Institute of Occupational Safety and Health (NIOSH), has estimated that 88 percent of those who work at computers three or more hours a day suffer from eyestrain, eye fatigue or glare-related headaches. CVS is very serious. It is pervasive … and it must be dealt with … the right way! Did you know that CVS is more common than Carpal Tunnel Syndrome?

In this chapter I am going to give you an overview of the unique characteristics of computers that make them so visually demanding and stressful, and helpful suggestions to improve your comfort. I even have a model workstation for you to copy. It has been shown that with the right computer workstation, companies that improved the ergonomics of their employees' workstation were able to see a 25 percent increase in employee productivity, a four to 19 percent increase in performance, less turnover of employees, and a decrease in error rates up to a factor of 15 times!

As I said before, when you are more comfortable, you will be more efficient, and therefore, a better employee. Let's get one thing straight right away. The unique characteristics and high visual demands of computer work will make many of us uncomfortable after prolonged periods in front of computers. In fact, it has been shown that the level of discomfort usually increases with the amount of computer use. The most common complaints are of headaches, blurred vision, and neck and shoulder pain. Whereas workers in other highly visually demanding occupations will also experience vision related symptoms, it is the unique characteristics and the high visual demands of computer work that makes the development of Computer Vision

Syndrome so prevalent. 88 percent of those who work at computers three or more hours a day have some form of Computer Vision Syndrome complaint. Viewing characters and images on a computer screen is different than viewing words on a piece of paper. Words on a page are two-dimensional. The letters on the cathode ray tube (CRT) computer screen are made-up of tiny pixels which are tiny flashes of light "floating" in space. Studies have shown that our eyes cannot focus on these pixel-generated characters with the same accuracy as words on a printed page. To add to this visual dilemma, the letters on a computer screen do not have the same sharply defined edges as printed letters on paper. Add to this the prevalence of screen glare and reduced contrast of the letters to the background, and one can start to realize that yes, viewing images on a computer screen is not an easy task for our visual systems. Remember, our human visual system is truly an amazing process and remarkably put together, but after many hours of computer work our eyes will "lose the battle" and start to have symptoms related to the prolonged stressful visual demands that computers impose upon our visual systems.

Computer work also demands that our viewing distances and viewing angles be different than those commonly used when we read, write or do other close activities. These differences also add to the stress of our visual systems while we perform computer work. These variations of our viewing distances and viewing angles sometimes necessitate the need for special computer or occupational eyewear.

The above examples highlight how stressful and visually demanding computer use is to our eyes. I have a lot of important information, suggestions and ideas to help you use a computer with much less eye and body fatigue. I have organized this into three main areas concerning computers. The three areas are monitors, lighting, and the ergonomics of your workstation. In each of these three, I have highlighted very easy-to-understand suggestions to help you achieve the most comfortable, efficient computer environment.

Your Monitor: Reading words on a monitor as compared to reading words on a printed page is much harder because of resolution, flicker and contrast. Resolution corresponds to the clarity of the characters (letters) produced by computer monitors. Computer characters are created by pixels, or electronically generated blocks of light, on the computer monitor. Unfortunately, those pixels produce characters with sloping margins instead of the true sharp edges that are common to words on a printed page. Were you to magnify the characters on a printed page and the computer's characters, you would see that the printed page's characters are generally more clearly produced. This decisively shows that the characters produced on a printed page have better resolution. Studies have shown that reading tasks were 20 to 30 percent slower on CRTs compared to a printed page; increased screen resolution has generally been shown to improve reading speed, reduce visual symptoms, or both. Greater pixel densities result in better performance and comfort.

The better the quality of your monitor and its resolution capability, the more you can improve your visual comfort and performance. It is my recommendation, then, to buy the highest quality display your budget allows. Flat panel displays or LCDs (Liquid Crystal Displays) are much more visually comfortable to our eyes than CRTs because they provide better contrast and do not flicker like the CRTs. LCDs create significantly less flicker which greatly reduces eyestrain. When the CRT display refreshes the characters, this causes the characters to "flicker." Although we may not actually "see" the characters refreshing or "flickering," studies have shown that our brain does respond to these imperceptible flickers and it does contribute to discomfort and decreased performance (efficiency).

Many computer users will feel uncomfortable with refresh rates of 60 Hz or even 70 Hz. The refresh rate of most CRT displays can be adjusted through software control panel settings. Although it is common for CRTs to have refresh rates in the 60 to 90 Hz range, I strongly recommend that you set the display to the highest refresh rate available. You can also decrease the discomfort associated with flicker by decreasing the display brightness.

Flicker, fortunately, is not a problem with LCDs. Flat panel displays are also much thinner because they do not have the bulky picture tube, helping to provide better workstation arrangements. For these reasons, I urge my patients, and you, to purchase only a flat panel or LCD monitor. Do not save your money on the CRT monitor. Save your eyes and purchase the more costly flat panel display. Period. No exceptions!

The size of the characters on the screen is very important for both function and comfort. How large should the characters on the screen be? This can be calculated by the *3X rule*. (This only applies to people 45 years old and younger who currently do not need reading glasses.) You should first measure your working distance (the distance from your eyes to the computer monitor). Next, multiply this distance by three. If you normally work with your eyes 24 inches from your computer screen, then you would multiply 24 by 3 and get 72 inches. Next, you should look at the characters on your screen from 72 inches away; the characters on the screen should still be discernible from there. If they are not, you should increase the size of the characters until they follow the 3X rule. This 3X rule is relatively simple to apply, and a must for anyone wishing to reduce computer eye strain. You can also determine the appropriate character size by backing away from the computer screen and noting the farthest distance at which you can just barely identify the characters on the screen. This is the threshold, and one-third of that distance represents the point at which the text is three times the threshold size; it also represents the maximum distance for you to be viewing the screen.

In our above example, if you could just discern the characters at 72 inches, then one-third of that distance, or 24 inches, would be the maximum viewing distance with that size character. (Again, this 3X rule only applies to persons under age 45 who do not yet require reading glasses and who are wearing the appropriate prescription when performing the test.)

Visual comfort on your computer monitor is also affected by the colors of the background and the characters on your computer screen. Dark backgrounds tend to create more reflection (glare) problems. It is usually best to have the brightness of the background of the screen match the brightness of the room. It is not comfortable for you to view a bright screen in a dark room, nor a dark screen in a bright room. Keeping the room, screen and documents at the same brightness is best for your visual comfort. Black characters on a white background is the best recommendation that I can give to you to achieve the best visual comfort at the computer. Dark backgrounds, as a general rule, would be the least visually comfortable, and studies have shown better performance with light backgrounds.

Lighting: Improper lighting is probably the most common environmental factor contributing to visual discomfort when working on a computer. This is often a case of too much light rather than too little light. When objects in the field of view have large differences in luminance (brightness), this contributes to significant discomfort. The most important principle of good lighting is to eliminate bright sources of light from the field of view and to achieve relatively even distribution of luminance (brightness) in the field of view.

When arranging or assessing your computer workstation, realize that overhead fluorescent lights emit their light in wide angles, resulting in light directly entering your eyes. Indirect lighting (ie: bouncing the light off the ceiling) will result in a more even distribution of light. Using a dark background computer display will usually result in a greater luminance disparity between the computer display and other objects in the room. Try to eliminate other areas where large luminance disparities are created. Windows not properly shaded, white paper on the desk, white desktop surfaces, and desk lamps aimed toward the eyes or that too highly illuminate the work area. Most of us do not pay enough attention to lighting, which is why it is often overlooked. However, improper or poorly designed lighting for your computer workstation creates a very stressful visual situation which will lead to discomfort and poor performance. Lighting has the ability to create a comfortable or uncomfortable computer workstation.

Windows can create a major source of glare. You will want to avoid facing an unshaded window since the difference in brightness between the computer screen and the area behind it may be extremely stressful and uncomfortable. Likewise, do not sit with your back to an unshaded window because it, too, will cause an uncomfortable computer workstation. All windows need to be properly shaded with curtains, blinds or adjustable shades. Sometimes, rearranging the workstation is necessary when a large window is causing discomfort glare.

The workstation needs to have a uniform brightness throughout. You cannot view a dark screen in a bright room, nor a bright screen in a dark room. You cannot have a bright task light and view a   dark screen. The lighting must be relatively even throughout. Why? Have you ever gone to a matinee at the movie theater? When you leave, the outside sunlight is blinding. This is what you are doing to your eyes, on a smaller scale, when you look at a dark screen and then a bright reference document. You are forcing your eyes to readjust to a new brightness level as you look back and forth from a dark object and then to a brighter object. Doing this repeatedly for long periods of time leads to a stressed-out visual system and eye fatigue. Remember, you want to make your eyes as comfortable as possible so that you can work for longer periods of time. That is the goal of this chapter!

Your immediate work area, that area on which your central vision is focused should not be very different in brightness from the rest of the room. The brightness of the central field should never be less than that of the surrounding area. In some cases where continuous, intense work is necessary, it can be slightly greater. Too great a contrast between the central and peripheral visual areas is uncomfortable and interferes with vision and work. A dark background on your monitor will dictate that the workstation lighting be less bright than if you use a brighter background on your display. The goal is to have the screen and the workstation lighting be as close in brightness (luminance) as possible. It has been found that most offices are two to three times as bright as they should be for computer use.

Glare is caused by a light source that is too bright or too close to the eyes or one that is positioned so that it reflects off surfaces in the work area. Bare light bulbs should never be used in a computer workstation environment. The brightness and position of lights should be adjusted to avoid glare, and shiny surfaces on furniture, walls, ceilings and other surfaces should be avoided. Remember that different colors will reflect light in different amounts. For example, black reflects only one percent of visible light, dark blue eight percent, light blue reflects 55 percent and light grey a staggering 75 percent!

Glare discomfort is caused by scattered light directly entering the eye. This is often caused by outside light or peripheral overhead lighting sources. This source of glare can be eliminated by using a visor or other shield to block out the light from the direction of the light. If the eyes feel better, then the light source is a problem which should be permanently addressed. One way to test for glare discomfort is to look at your computer screen and notice if there are any bright lights visible in your peripheral field. You can use your hand or a file folder to shield your eyes like a baseball cap visor to see if this gives you an improvement in comfort. Whether glare is from a window or an overhead fluorescent lighting, an immediate sense of visual comfort will help you to locate unwanted glare sources. Now here is an important piece of information for you to keep in mind the next time you visit the computer store. Glare guards and other "cutesy" devices that computer store salesmen want you to buy are not the key. Proper lighting at and around your workstation is far more critical. (I do, however, recommend glare guards endorsed by the American Optometric Association (AOA) if you have a CRT computer monitor).

Ergonomics and Your Workstation: It is widely recognized that "the eyes lead the body." Because working at the computer is such a visually intensive task, our body will do whatever is necessary to get our eyes into a visually comfortable and efficient position, often at the expense of good posture, resulting in musculoskeletal ailments such as a sore neck and shoulders.

Research suggests that longer viewing distances tend to be more visually comfortable. Longer viewing distances place less demand on the eyes to turn in (converge) and focus. A slightly downward viewing angle has also been shown to be more comfortable. This, too, is easier for the eyes, as it is known that it is easier for our eyes to converge when we look slightly downward. (Think about this: when you read a book do you hold the book straight out in front of you, or do you hold the book lower than straight ahead? You tend to hold the book low and look downward when reading. This is because it is naturally easier and more comfortable for your eyes to look downward when looking at something close). Studies support this, clearly indicating better performance and comfort with ocular depression (downward gaze) compared to elevation (upward gaze). For typical computer viewing distances, an ocular depression angle (downward gaze) of 10 to 20 degrees relative to straight-ahead gaze (horizontal plane) seems indicated for optimal performance and comfort. Although there can be considerable differences between computer users regarding their preferred elevation and viewing distances, studies have further shown peak performance with 10 degrees of depression (downward gaze), and comfort was best with 10 to 20 degrees of downward gaze.

As for the height of the monitor, most of our body's adaptation is accomplished at the neck. If the computer display is located too high, most people tilt their head back so that they can maintain the usual and more comfortable downward viewing angle. This postural adjustment to a higher screen can cause neck and back aches. A monitor that is placed so that the primary viewing angle is horizontal or straight ahead is considered to be too high. Remember, the preferred or most comfortable gaze angle is slightly downward. A monitor placed too high will also tend to increase discomfort glare. The higher the monitor, the more upward you look, the wider your eyes will be open, and this will lead to drier eyes (your tears will evaporate more quickly). Therefore, a monitor that is too high will increase ocular discomfort of your convergence system, increase glare discomfort and increase dry eyes. A monitor can also be improperly positioned too low. A monitor positioned too low will cause forward flexion of the torso and neck. This in turn, will cause neck and back aches. A low monitor will usually cause computer users to support some of their body weight with their arms, potentially creating wrist problems, as well. As previously stated, the monitor should be positioned below the horizontal plane of the eyes at straight-ahead gaze. This will not only be optimal for your visual system, but in turn (because the eyes lead the body) optimal for your neck and back, as well. In order to achieve the recommended 10 to 20 degrees of downward gaze, a good rule of thumb is to set up your workstation so that the top of the monitor is at or slightly below eye level.

At what angle should the screen be tilted? Although there is little research in this area, I will recommend two common sense approaches to this question. When you read a book or magazine, you hold it so that the top is not perpendicular to your line of sight, but so that the top is slightly tilted away from perpendicular (or away from you). Therefore, recommendation number one would be to position the screen so that the top is tilted slightly away from you.

My second recommendation would be to position the screen so that it eliminates or reduces any reflections or glare. If the tilt gives you a comfortable viewing angle, then that is the right tilt for you and your vision dynamics.

Central to any good computer workstation is that you place whatever you view most often during your workday straight in front of you. Whatever you look at the most, be it your monitor, your reference material, or something else during your time at your workstation, it is a *must* that it be placed *straight in front of you!* You would be surprised to find out how many people set up their workstations so that they are looking mostly off to one side during their time at their workstation!

The location of the reference material is also very critical. Many people will place the computer monitor straight in front of them, and then put the reference documents on the table next to the screen. This is a no-no! It is not very efficient; this will cause you to make large and frequent eye, head and upper torso movements to look back and forth from the reference documents to the screen. An easy way to solve this problem is to purchase a copyholder so that you can place the reference documents next to the computer monitor. Another solution can be to place the reference document so that it is between the computer monitor and the keyboard. Remember, you want to decrease unnecessary frequent and repetitive eye, head, neck and torso movements.

Workstation Set-up: The illustration on the accompanying page shows the ideal workstation set-up, as recommended by the American Optometric Association (AOA). Although this set-up seems to be the least stressful on the body, no body position (posture) is ideal for long periods of time. The neck, back, shoulder and wrist pains common to computer users is most likely the result of sitting in one position for long periods of time without shifting body positions or getting up and taking regular breaks. When designing a computer workstation, we start from the ground up. The descriptions below should help to clarify and further enhance your understanding of the illustration.

Chair: A proper task chair is the starting point. The correct chair and its adjustment will have the following:

- *Legs/rollers* – five legs are recommended (fewer legs are less stable and can possibly tip over).
- *Height adjustment* – the chair should have an adjustable height capability. The height of the chair should be adjusted so that your feet are firmly on the floor, with your thighs evenly supported on the seat pan, and the angle at the knee should be slightly greater than 90 degrees (i.e., your thigh should be oriented slightly downward from the hip to the knee). A footrest may be required to allow the chair to be adjusted higher.
- *Back support* – Back support is critical, especially lower back support. If your chair has an adjustable lower back support, adjust it for your height. If your chair does not support your lower back sufficiently, I urge you to consider purchasing an ergonomic cushion.
- *Back tilt* – if your chair has a back tilt adjustment, you should adjust it so that your upper torso is tipped slightly back (i.e., away from the monitor).
- *Tilt tension* – the tilt tension should be adjusted so that you are in a firm upright position. The chair should not tilt or rock backward too easily; -this can lead to poor posture, and especially neck strain.
- *Armrests* – your chair *must* be fitted with arm-

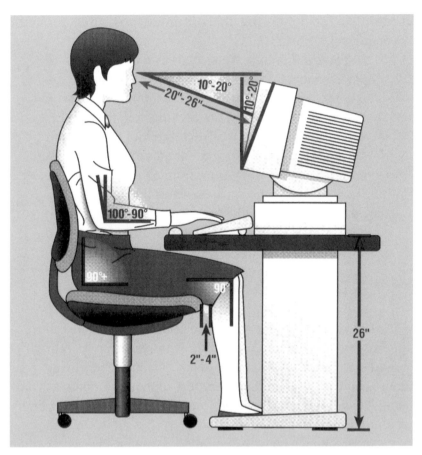

rests. Without armrests, the unsupported arms tend to cause a sore neck and shoulders. Wrist problems can also develop from supporting your arms' weight with your wrists on the top. Proper armrests should have soft, rounded edges and should be able to be adjusted in and out, and up and down. Properly adjusted armrests should support the elbows, forearms, or both can be supported while typing.

Keyboard & wrists: The placement of the computer keyboard in relation to our hands and wrists has a direct effect on the comfort our bodies and, hence, the comfort of our eyes. Following are guidelines for achieving the optimum positions for both keyboard and wrists.

- *Keyboard Positioning* – the keyboard should be placed directly in front of the body so the hands can fall into the proper position of the left index finger on the "f" key and the right index finger on the "j" key.
- *Keyboard Height* – adjust the height of your keyboard (if possible) so that your forearm is oriented slightly downward from elbow to wrist.
- *Wrist Angle* – the most comfortable position for our wrists is straight (i.e., no right or left bend) and extended 0 to 20 degrees upward. Using a soft wrist rest in front of the keyboard is usually helpful. As mentioned above, armrests should be adjusted to provide comfortable support for your elbows and forearms to achieve the proper wrist angle.

Mouse: Your mouse should be located immediately next to your keyboard so that you don't have to reach for it. Your wrist should not rest heavily on the desk surface when using your mouse. As with the keyboard, armrest support is important when using your mouse. An external or wireless mouse is strongly recommended when using a laptop.

Copyholder: A copyholder should be used whenever possible. The copyholder will allow you to locate your reference documents close to your computer monitor so that you can avoid excessive head, neck, and even upper torso movement.

Computer monitor: The proper height of your computer monitor should be placed so that you are looking downward approximately 10 to 20 degrees. The top of the computer monitor should be at or slightly below eye level.

Set up your computer workstation following the above guidelines, and you will be well on your way toward reducing the detrimental effects of computer use on your vision.

Chapter Seven:
The Issue of Corrective Lenses

Author's Note: It's me, nagging you once again, for your own good – now is the time to rest your eyes! So go ahead and practice your two minute break before reading on..

Perhaps the previous chapters have helped to give you an understanding of how stressful the visual demands of our information society is to our visual systems. Moreover, I hope you have learned a bit of useful information about how you can be your eyes' own best friend when it comes to avoiding damage to your visual system from the stress of computer use.

We adults are using computers more frequently and for more hours in each workday, but it is our children that I am most concerned with. The near-point demands (reading and computer work – GameBoy® and PSP® included) that our children face is an ever-growing and serious problem. As an optometrist, I find myself having to regularly increase the prescriptions for my young myopic patients in order for them to see as well as they did the year before. Many college students return to me every May and June, complaining of poor vision after a visually demanding year at school.

Whereas newer eye surgical procedures, such as LASIK, are temporarily reducing our patient base, the large percentage of children now wearing distance vision correction is more than making up for it. I believe I am accurate in telling my patients that over 50 percent of children (in good academic towns) will probably wear eyeglasses or contact lenses by age 16. This, in my view, is a major shift in the eyeglass-wearing population. Although the word "epidemic" might be too strong and too alarming, please realize that *most children* will need to wear glasses by age 16 and certainly many more will by the age of 25!

If you are an adult over age 30 and you are reading this, think back to your younger days and try to recall all the children back then who were wearing glasses in grade school and even in high school. I will bet your recall is going to remind you that *most* of the children back then *did not* wear eyeglasses or contact lenses. Think about this: the new generation of children is not the same, nor is genetics causing this situation, but rather it is the huge amounts of time that our children are spending in visually demanding near-oriented activities for prolonged periods of time!

This is why I try to reassure the parents of my young patients that, even though their children's eyes are continuing to change annually (and in many cases much sooner), these young patients' eyes are healthy. I do *not* encourage them to have their children avoid reading, but I do encourage frequent rest breaks and limiting leisure time on the computer and video games. I do tell them that smart people wear glasses (from studying a lot), and that I would rather that they have "thick glasses and a thick brain, than no glasses and no brain!"

Another way to slow or stop the nearsighted progression of children and adults (besides avoiding long periods of computer use, reading and other nearpoint tasks) is to wear rigid gas permeable contact lenses (RGPs). These are the newer generation of "hard" contact lenses. The advantage to wearing soft contact lenses is convenience and initial comfort. RGPs can take up to two weeks to be comfortable; soft contact lenses are usually comfortable within three minutes. RGPs will usually give better vision than soft contact lenses and there is greater oxygen transmissibility to the cornea when wearing RGPs. The only other downside with RGPs is that if any dust or dirt gets under the lens, the wearer will experience major discomfort. I personally most often fit soft contact lenses because my patient population is looking for immediate comfort and the convenience that only soft contact lenses can offer them. I have, in fact, started with RGPs instead of soft contact lenses. They were not comfortable with the RGPs and instead chose to return to conventional eyeglasses. It is really a hard decision to make, to be sure. The soft contact lenses will allow your child to be comfortable and smiling day one, but in the long run, the RGPs will probably control the nearsighted progression. In fact, many optometrists are actually re-shaping patients' corneas with RGPs in order to reduce nearsightedness. When employed correctly, these RGPs can often *reduce* your eyeglass prescription. If you have a lower powered lens prescription (usually -4.00 Diopters or less) it is possible to reduce your prescription to the point where you no longer will need to wear eyeglasses or contact lenses during the day. An RGP is still usually worn during sleep as a "retainer" to maintain your prescription at the new level.

Epilogue

Author's Note: *Last time – I promise – now get busy and do your two minute break. Your eyes are going to thank you.*

Computers, deskwork, reading and other prolonged near-point activities are here to stay. There is no escaping that fact. We live in an information society, and our culture demands that we perform these activities on a regular basis. Almost every civilized person must do extended nearpoint tasks on a some-what regular, if not daily basis.

As I have said before, don't change your job – *change your habits*. I do not want children to avoid reading or studying. Instead, I recommend that they take frequent rest breaks and not spend hours of their leisure time in front of computers or playing those highly stressful video games.

I have given you specific exercises and changes of habits advice in previous chapters. Below, I just want to remind you and reiterate the most important, simple steps that each of you must *(and can easily)* do.

Any prolonged nearpoint activity requires frequent rest breaks. After 15 minutes of nearpoint activity (reading, computer, video gaming, hobby work, etc.), you must stop and look far away *for a full two minutes*. Relax. Take these two minute rest breaks *every 15 minutes*. Then after one hour of the activity, *stop,* get up, get yourself a drink of water, go to the bathroom – *whatever*. You must physically get up and move! *Don't just sit there* for more than one hour straight – you must physically stand up and move around.

For nearpoint activities that require you to sit for more than one hour, consider doing some of the eye exercises (near-far rock, rotations, etc.) that I have previously described. Also, don't be afraid to go that "extra mile" with a good stretch and movement of your other body parts – legs, arms, shoulders, etc. It is not natural for humans to remain in one position for prolonged periods of time. *Move your body regularly.*

For the frequent computer user for whom this book has been written, I want to reiterate some primary recommendations:

- The computer monitor must be lower than straight ahead, and absolutely not high so that you are looking upward. Setting up your monitor so that you are looking 10 to 20 degrees downward is ideal. (A good rule of thumb is such that the top of the monitor is at or slightly below eye level).
- Consciously blink your eyes. (Remember that a good blink is to close your eyes softly and gently, keeping them closed for two to three seconds.) Studies show that computer users tend to stare at their monitors and blink about 50 to 80 percent less than normal blink rates. *Blink frequently!*
- The lighting at your workstation needs to be as even as possible. Do not have a dark screen in a bright room, nor a bright screen in a dark room. Do not have a bright task light and then look at a dark screen. The lighting should be as even as possible.
- Eliminate all sources of glare. Windows need to be shaded. There should be no bright lights in your peripheral view.
- If you do not have a flat screen, but instead have the older CRT screen, set your refresh rate at the highest possible setting. Also, use a glare guard that has the American Optometric Association's (AOA) Seal of Acceptance.
- If you are wearing bifocals, I do not recommend you wear your everyday bifocals at your computer workstation. Your everyday bifocals are made so that the top part of the bifocal allows you to see

clearly at 20 feet and further; the bottom of your bifocal is made for you to read at about 16 inches. When looking through the top of your bifocals, your computer is obviously not 20 feet away. If you try to look through the bottom part, you will *constantly have to lift your head,* definitely *leading to neck strain.* Don't do this! *If you have progressive addition lenses* (no-line multifocal lenses), these can work if you are able to set up your monitor so that it is very low and a little further than would be normal. (This will give you an opportunity to use the intermediate or lower part of the lens as you gaze downward towards the monitor). The narrow intermediate zone of progressive addition lenses are not ideal, but if they allow you to see clearly and comfortably, they can be used. The *best* option for you is to set up your workstation and monitor so you are able to use a *single vision eyeglass lens* (not bifocal or progressive) that will give you clear, comfortable vision to your keyboard, work area and monitor. If this is not possible due to the way your monitor and workstation are arranged, I also like a bifocal made just for your computer workstation or *no-line computer-only eyeglasses* with lenses designed exclusively for your workstation. Such lenses are usually called computer lens or occupational lens designs. They are specially designed for a computer workstation environment. Some of the more popular lenses in this group are AO Technica®, Cosmolit Office®, Essilor Interview®, Hoya Tact®, Shamir Office®, SOLA Access® and Zeiss Gradel RD®.

When it comes to your eyewear choices, be it soft contact lenses, rigid gas permeable contact lenses or eyeglasses, common sense is a must. Contact lenses do not naturally occur in your eyes. They are foreign objects introduced into the eye. As such, realize that they cannot allow as much oxygen to our corneas as would nothing at all. (Even though the new silicone hydrogel soft contact lenses have been approved for up to 30 continuous days of uninterrupted wear, I still do not recommend that my patients regularly sleep with them). They also can trap debris and other substances below them and cause problems. They can rip, tear, break, chip and cause corneal abrasions. The reduced oxygen supply to the cornea can lead to infections and other problems. *Practice moderation!*

I recommend you never deliberately sleep with contact lenses (except the corneal reshaping RGPs). Take out your lenses for a minimum of 2 hours each day. Practice the moderation recommended in the chapter on corrective lenses and, as is the case with anything in life, you will be doing what is best for you. Wear eyeglasses every day. I often say to my patients, "You don't have to be seen in public wearing your eyeglasses – just wear them in the house for two hours or more each day. It is better to wear your eyeglasses in your house for two hours than to get an infection and be forced to wear your eyeglasses all day for two weeks until your infection is gone."

I hope this all makes sense to you. After all, just like the rest of this book, it is *basic common sense for healthy vision.*

Acknowledgments

This book has been a "work in progress" for over 15 years. Its ideas were founded in the summer of 1988, when at the age of 22 I lost my "perfect" 20/20 vision. I was working at a summer job that demanded I read for eight to nine hours each day, Monday through Friday. By the end of the summer, I had become slightly nearsighted from the intense reading demands of my job. That fall, I entered optometry school and learned many principles and theories on how the muscles in our eyes work when we read and perform close activities. I learned that if I had never read for all those hours five days a week at my summer job, I would more than likely *still have* that perfect vision I had previously enjoyed my first 22 years of life. Through my studies and my clinical experience I have fine-tuned and revised my theories on the effect of prolonged reading and close activities on our visual systems and, particularly, on the progression of nearsightedness.

I would like to thank my father, Dr. E. Michael Geiger (also an optometrist and author), for all his help in getting my ideas into print and in the correct language for my peers, patients and all those interested in nearsighted progression from prolonged nearpoint activities. I would also like to acknowledge and thank Dr. James Sheedy and Dr. Peter G. Shaw-McMinn for allowing me to use much of their computer knowledge from their book, *Diagnosing and Treating Computer-Related Vision Problems*. Dr. James Sheedy is the nation's leading authority on computers and the eyes. I urge all my readers to explore his truly informative website at www.doctorergo.com.

Lastly, I wish to acknowledge and thank my wife, Audrey, and our daughter, Hayley, for all their support and love during this important project and time in my life.

Bibliography

Anshel, J., *Visual Ergonomics in the Workplace*, Taylor & Francis, 1998.

Anshel, J., "The CVS Epidemic. How You Can Make Computers Easier on the Eyes," *Review of Optometry*, May 1999; 136 (5).

Bates, W., *The Bates Method for Better Eyesight Without Glasses*, Henry Holt, 1981.

Beresford, S., Muris, D., Allen, M., Young, F., *Improve Your Vision Without Glasses or Contact Lenses*, Fireside, 1996.

Bommarito, P., "The CVS Epidemic. Your Role in Easing the Aches and Pains of Computer Users," *Review of Optometry*, July 1999; 136 (7).

Corbett, M., *Help Yourself to Better Eyesight,* Prentice-Hall, 1949.

Donnenfeld, E., Thimons, J.J., "The CVS Epidemic. How to Ease the Symptoms of Dry Eye in Computer Users," *Review of Optometry*, June 1999; 136 (6).

Kinney, J., Laria, S., Ryan, A., et al. "The Vision of Submariners and National Guardsmen: A Longitudinal Study," *American Journal of Optometry and Physiology*. October, 1980; 57: 469-478.

Osias, G., "The CVS Epidemic: Part IV. You Have the Cure, So Let Patients Know It," *Review of Optometry,* August 1999; 136 (8).

Quackenbush, T., *Relearning to See*, North Atlantic Books, 1999.

Rehm, D., *The Myopia Myth*, International Myopia Prevention Association, 1981.

Schneider, M., *Yoga for Your Eyes*, Sounds True, 1999.

Sheedy, J., Shaw-McMinn, P., *Diagnosing and Treating Computer-Related Vision Problems,* Butterworth-Heinemann, 2003.

Young, F., "Primate Myopia," *The American Journal of Optometry and Archives of the American Academy of Optometry*, 1981; 58 (7): 560-566.

Young, F., "The Development and Retention of Myopia by Monkeys," *The American Journal of Optometry and Archives of the American Academy of Optometry*, 1961; 38 (10): 545-555.

Young, F., et al, "The Transmission of Refractive Errors within Eskimo Families," *The American Journal of Optometry and Archives of the American Academy of Optometry*, 1969; 46 (9).

About the Author

Dr. Kevin D. Geiger, O.D.

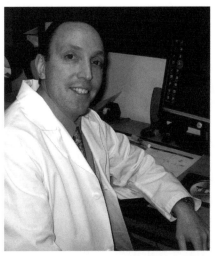

Dr. Geiger received his doctor of optometry degree from the State University of New York, State College of Optometry. He has held the position of Director of the Alumni Association since 1992.

Dr. Geiger is a practicing optometrist with offices in Manalapan and Livingston, New Jersey, as well as Staten Island, New York. He is the past recipient of the Frederick Brock Memorial Award for his clinical expertise in working with patients requiring vision therapy and other visual interventions for a multitude of ocular conditions relating to binocular and perceptual deficiencies. He is one of only six optometrists in the State of New Jersey to be recognized as a "Computer Vision Syndrome" specialist, after completing additional education in the area of computers and their effects on the visual system.

He resides with his wife and daughter in Marlboro, New Jersey. Always seeking knowledge and to better himself, Dr. Geiger is an avid reader of literature dealing with nutrition, vitamins and alternative medicine. He is also past Vice President of the Freehold Phrasers chapter of Toastmasters International.

Other Books by Safe Goods Publishing

	$ US	$ CAN
The ADD and ADHD Diet	9.95	14.95
ADD, The Natural Approach	4.95	6.95
Testosterone is your Friend	8.95	12.95
Eye Care Naturally	8.95	12.95
The Natural Prostate Cure	6.95	10.95
Zen Macrobiotics for Americans	7.95	11.95
Kids-First: Health with No Interference*	16.95	24.95
The Minerals You Need	4.95	6.95
Cancer Disarmed Expanded	7.95	11.95
What is Beta Glucan	4.95	6.95
Overcoming Senior Moments	7.95	11.95
No More Horse Estrogen	7.95	11.95
Live Disease Free	9.95	14.95
The Secrets of Staying Young	9.95	14.95
2012 Airborne Prophesy	16.95	24.95
Atlantis Today - The USA	9.95	14.95
Analyzing Sports Drinks	4.95	6.95

*Newly expanded edition

For a complete listing of books visit our web site:
www.safegoodspub.com to order or call (888) 628-8731
for a free catalog (888) NATURE-1